IRISH TERRIER DOG

The Complete Handbook On How To Raising And Caring For Irish Terrier Dog

CHAD BRUNO

Table of Contents

Introductory

The Irish terrier is a type of dog that was first developed in that country. The breed is well-known for its unique physical and behavioral characteristics. For a quick definition of Irish terrier, consider the following:

• Irish Terriers, often called Irish Red Terriers, can be traced back to the Emerald Isle. They were developed for their hunting and rodent-control abilities, as well as their guarding and social abilities.

• Irish Terriers are medium-sized canines with a wiry coat with red or wheaten tones. They seem very different from other animals and are rather attractive. They are somewhat protected from the elements by their dense, straight, and tough coat.

• Irish Terriers have an outspoken, self-assured, and energetic temperament. They are known to be good-natured and friendly in addition to being intelligent and loyal. Brave and fearless, these dogs have earned the nickname "daredevils."

• Irish Terriers have a long history of service as hunting companions, especially for small wildlife such as rats, foxes, and otters. Farms also used them as security dogs. Because of their amiable and devoted temperament, they are primarily kept as pets in modern times.

• Irish Terriers are smart dogs, but they also have a strong personality and may be difficult to train. In order to channel their energy and stubbornness into constructive activities, they need early socialization and persistent, positive reinforcement training.

• Because of their high energy levels, Irish Terriers need regular physical activity to thrive. Boredom can be avoided by regular exercise, fun, and mental stimulation.

• Maintenance they need frequent brushing to keep their wiry coat from matting and looking its best. Their coat may require occasional hand-stripping (the removal of dead hair).

• **Health:** Like any breeds, Irish Terriers are prone to various health conditions, including hip dysplasia, thyroid disorders, and allergies. Their health relies on responsible breeding and regular trips to the vet.

In conclusion, the Irish Terrier is a type of dog native to Ireland that has historically served as a hunting and guarding companion. When raised and socialized properly, they can make devoted pets for their owners.

CHAPTER ONE
Learning about Irish Terriers

There are several facets to the Irish Terrier that must be taken into account if one is to gain a comprehensive understanding of the breed. **Here is a complete rundown of the Irish Terrier:**

• Originating in what is now Ireland, the Irish Terrier is one of the first terrier breeds. They were developed to pursue rodents, otters, and foxes, among other tiny prey. These canines also served as guard dogs and farm helpers. They were prized for their bravery, tenacity, and hunting prowess, all of which contributed to the breed's reputation and success in the workplace.

Outer Description:

• Male Irish Terriers normally weigh 25 to 27 pounds (11 to 12 kg), while females tend to be a little smaller.

• **Coat:** Their coats range in color from brilliant red to wheaten, and are dense, wiry, and rough. This unique coat is a defense against the elements and predators.

• **Body:** They have a well-proportioned, compact body with a straight back, deep chest, and a powerful, muscular build. In some nations, the docking of their tails is legal, although this is changing.

- **Head:** Irish Terriers have a narrow head with a long, flat skull, short V-shaped ears, and dark, expressive eyes.

- Irish Terriers' temperament is recognized for being lively and friendly.

They are fearless and refuse to back down from any confrontation.

- Terriers are known for their loyalty and devotion to their owners.

They are an active breed that needs daily walks and mental games to stay happy.

• These dogs are bright, but they also tend to be stubborn, so consistent training is essential.

Necessary Maintenance:

• Physical activity: Irish Terriers require regular physical activity to release excess energy. All pets need regular exercise, fun activities, and access to a safe yard.

Strong-willed dogs need early socialization and obedience training to keep them in check.

To keep its texture and prevent matting, a rough coat needs to be brushed and hand-stripped regularly.

• **Health:** Regular vet check-ups are vital to manage their health, as with any breed. Because of the potential for some health problems, finding a reputable breeder is essential.

• **Suitable Owners:** Irish Terriers are a perfect match for energetic adults or families that can offer them with both physical and mental stimulation. They do best in a warm, structured setting with lots of human company.

Finally, the Irish Terrier is a breed that is full of life and bravery, with a long tradition of hunting and undying loyalty. Anyone thinking about getting one of these dogs as a companion would do well to learn as much as possible about their background, appearance, personality, needs, and care. Irish Terriers need to be kept in good health, so responsible breeding and care are essential.

Locating a Trustworthy Adoption Center or Breeder

When looking to adopt or purchase a dog of any breed, it is essential to undertake research to find a reliable breeder or rescue group. Find an ethical Irish Terrier breeder or rescue organization by following these suggestions.

1. Trustworthy Breeder:

a. Irish Terrier Club of America or whatever its official name is in your country. These groups frequently compile lists of breeders and promote those they deem to be ethical operators.

b. Reputable breeders can be found in online databases and directories. Try visiting kennel club websites or researching breed-specific websites. It's best to exercise caution with breeders who rely heavily on posting ads in online classifieds.

c. You can get referrals from people you know, such as other Irish Terrier owners, doctors, and dog trainers. Word of mouth recommendations from those you trust can be extremely helpful.

d. When looking for a reliable breeder, you should ask them the following questions to verify their legitimacy:

Is the place where the puppies are being raised sanitary?

• Can you meet the puppy's parents or at least one of them?

Do the breeding dogs come with proof of good health?

How have the puppies been handled and trained?

• Do they have recommendations from people who have purchased puppies from them in the past?

To what extent do they vaccinate and deworm their puppies?

Does the breeder and buyer have a written agreement outlining their respective responsibilities?

Do they have breed expertise and time to offer advice and assistance?

2. Groups That Help Save People:

a. Find Irish Terrier-specific rescue groups by doing an online search. They frequently have adoptable dogs. You can search for adoptable Irish Terriers in your region on websites like Petfinder and Adopt-a-Pet.

b. Visit your local animal shelter and ask if they have any Irish Terriers or terrier mixes available for adoption. It is possible to find adoptable purebred dogs at animal shelters.

c. Online Dog Adoption Platforms: Research various online resources that have canine adoption listings. Don't forget to check out the profiles and reach out to the rescue groups for more details.

d. Learn about the steps involved in adopting a child, which often include filling out paperwork, having a home visit, and paying a cost. Verify that the rescue group offers adequate help and follow-up, and that you are ready to take on the duties of dog ownership.

Factors to Think About

• If at all possible, go to the breeder's or rescue's location to see the dogs in person and get a feel for the environment.

• If a breeder or rescue organization has warning signs like not disclosing health information, having unclean facilities, or not letting you meet the dogs, you should proceed with caution.

Do your homework on the breed to make sure it suits your needs.

• Be prepared to provide a loving and stable home for your Irish Terrier.

A dog is a lifelong companion, therefore it's important to find a breeder or shelter that cares about their well-being. A respectable breeder or rescue group will supply you with a healthy, well-socialized Irish Terrier and offer help throughout the dog's life.

CHAPTER TWO
The Basics of Irish Terrier Care

Keeping an Irish Terrier in good health is crucial to ensuring their happiness. When caring for this breed, keep these things in mind regarding their health:

1. Veterinarian Checkups:

To keep an eye on your Irish Terrier's health and head off any problems in their tracks, you should take him or her in for checkups on a regular basis.

Vaccinate regularly and take any preventative measures advised by your veterinarian.

2. Nutrition:

• Offer a premium dog food that is tailored to the specific nutritional requirements of Irish Terriers.

As these canines tend toward obesity, careful portion management is essential.

3. Exercise:

• Irish Terriers, being an energetic breed, need regular physical and mental stimulation in the form of exercise.

• Walk, play, or engage in some other sort of physical activity for at least 30-60 minutes daily.

4. Grooming:

Maintaining the coat and the general cleanliness of your Irish Terrier requires regular grooming sessions.

To keep their wiry coat from matting and to eliminate any dead hair, you should brush it often.

• Their coat's texture may require regular hand-stripping, a method of removing dead hair.

5. Oral Health:

To avoid dental problems like plaque and tartar accumulation, you should routinely brush your dog's teeth.

Oral hygiene aids like dental chews and toys are also available.

6. Managing Parasites:

• Protect your dog from parasites like fleas, ticks, and worms. For the best preventative care options, talk to your vet.

• Always inspect your dog for ticks and other external parasites after going outside, but especially before bringing him within.

7. Checkups and Exams:

• Irish Terriers can be prone to specific inherited health concerns. Think about getting checked for things like hypothyroidism, eye problems, and hip dysplasia.

• The parents of the dog should have health clearances, which a reputable breeder should offer.

8. Spaying/Neutering:

• Talk to your vet about when it's best to spay or neuter your Irish Terrier. Their future health and behavior may be affected.

9. Allergies:

• Irish terriers can have skin allergies just like humans. See a doctor for diagnosis and treatment of allergies if your dog shows any symptoms (such as scratching, redness, or irritation).

10. Character and Psychological Well-Being:

• Irish Terriers are pack animals who benefit greatly from human interaction. Avoid boredom by spending quality time with your dog and challenging his mind with new experiences.

11. Recognize the Symptoms of Illness

• Familiarize yourself with the usual indicators of disease in dogs, such as changes in food, energy level, or behavior, and see your vet if you observe any alarming symptoms.

12. Disaster Preparation:

• Be prepared for unexpected events by knowing basic canine first aid and having access to a 24-hour veterinarian clinic.

13. Breeding with care:

• Choose a reputable breeder that invests in their dogs' health and happiness if you want to bring home an Irish Terrier from a litter.

If you give your Irish Terrier the care they need, they should live a long and happy life with you. Regular veterinarian care, correct feeding, exercise, grooming, and attention to their individual needs are crucial to keeping this breed happy and healthy.

Learning the Rules of Obedience

Training in basic obedience will help your Irish Terrier to become a well-mannered, secure, and enjoyable companion.

1. Sit:

• Raise a tasty reward high above your dog's head.

• Your dog will sit down naturally as its head tilts back to follow the treat. Give them the goodie and praise them when they sit.

• While they are sitting, say the word "sit" as a verbal cue. Slowly but surely, the two will become inextricably linked in their minds.

2. Stay:

• Have your dog sit down first.

Hold your hand out with the palm facing your dog and say "stay."

• Back up a little bit. If your dog stays put, praise and reward them.

As your dog gains experience and proficiency, you should extend the walks and hikes together.

3. Lay Flat:

• Have your dog sit down first.

Hold a reward close to your dog's nose and slowly lower it to the floor while saying "down."

You should praise and encourage your dog as soon as it lays down after following the treat.

4. Remember (Come):

• Keep your dog in a secure, contained location with a long leash.

Reduce your height to theirs, say their name, and tell them to "come."

• Pull the leash gently to call them over.

Encourage and reward them when they get to you. The leash should be used at an increasingly farther distance.

5. Put It Away:

• Exhibit a goodie in your hand and encourage your dog to approach.

Say "leave it" and put your hand over your fist.

• If your dog stops pulling away from the goodie and stops attempting to reach it, open your hand and give them a different treat.

6. Walking at a Heel (or on a Very Loose Leash)

• Initiate leashed walks with your dog. Keep your hand on the leash loosely.

To have your dog walk along you, use the word "heel" as a command.

• Praise your dog when he or she is well-behaved and walking loosely with you. Wait until they are back by your side to continue walking if they pull.

7. Keep seated and don't move:

• To use these commands, the "down" or "sit" command is combined with the word "stay."

• Once your dog understands "down" and "sit," start having it hold those positions for longer and farther apart.

Educating Hints:

• Reward your dog for good behavior with positive reinforcement like treats, praise, and affection.

• Keep training sessions short (10-15 minutes) and end on a good note.

• Maintain uniformity in your instructions and requirements.

Commands should be practiced in a variety of settings.

Patience is essential. It's important to go at your dog's pace, as not all canines learn at the same rate.

• Never resort to physical force or harsh punishment when teaching your dog; this can damage your relationship with him.

If you're new to dog training or run into problems, it may be helpful to take a basic obedience lesson taught by a professional dog trainer. Training your Irish Terrier will not only make them a well-behaved companion but also enhance your bond with them.

Providing your Irish Terrier with mental stimulation and enrichment is essential to his health. Keeping your dog busy with these pursuits is a great way

to ensure their mental and emotional well-being. Some suggestions for giving your Irish Terrier a stimulating mental environment:

1. Game of Clue:

• Toys that require your dog to use his or her brain should be used, such as puzzle toys and toys that dispense goodies. Their ability to think critically will be put to use.

2. Hide-and-Seek:

• Hide toys or treats and send your dog on a treasure hunt throughout the house. This satisfies their innate drive to hunt and provides a welcome mental challenge.

3. Direction & Instructions:

• Continue training sessions beyond basic obedience. You can keep your dog mentally stimulated by teaching it new tricks and commands.

4. You should do scent work with your Irish Terrier. Have them use their excellent sense of smell to sniff out hidden rewards and scented items.

5. Agility:

• Make a mini agility course for your dog in the backyard or nearby park. Any combination of hurdles, tunnels, and weave poles is fair game. Your dog's physical and mental abilities will be tested throughout agility training.

6. Socialization:

• Expose your Irish Terrier to new people, other animals, and settings on a regular basis. Regular interaction with others helps them maintain cognitive flexibility.

7. Playdates:

• You should set up doggie play dates. Dogs pick up useful information from one another and take part in challenging mental games.

8. Obstacles to Obedience:

• Put your dog's obedience to the test by having them "stay" while you hide, then calling them to come find you. This presents a novel mental challenge to the traditional recall instruction.

9. Games That Give Out Food:

• Put peanut butter, biscuits, or dog food into a frozen Kong and use it as a puzzle toy. This is great for your brain and body.

10. Curious & Unusual Stuff:

• Keep your dog interested by providing him with novel objects and games. Don't let them get bored with their toys by switching them out regularly.

11. Tune in and watch:

• Some canines benefit from the combination of enjoyment and mental stimulation provided by listening to soothing music or watching dog-themed television shows.

12. Reinforcement Learning:

• When your dog participates in mentally challenging activities, be sure to praise, treat, and reinforce him with positive reinforcement. This inspires people to seek out new information and knowledge.

13. Mind Exercises:

• Get or make some dog-friendly puzzles and logic games. The games need analytical and problem-solving skills.

14. Home Improvements:

• Using cardboard boxes, plastic bottles, and other non-hazardous household items, you may make your own puzzles and toys.

15. Education Programs:

• Structured cerebral stimulation can be achieved through enrolling your Irish Terrier in advanced training classes like agility or obedience competitions.

Never forget that your dog is an individual, and his or her mental stimulation needs should reflect that. Pay close attention to your Irish Terrier so you may tailor their mental enrichment to their own interests. A intellectually engaged and happy dog is more likely to be well-behaved and content.

CHAPTER THREE
Advancement and Expansion

It's crucial for the health and happiness of a new Irish Terrier puppy to know what to expect as they mature. Here is a rundown of the typical ages at which Irish Terriers go through each stage of development:

1. Age of the Newborn (0–2 Weeks):

• Puppies of the Irish Terrier breed are at this stage of their development. They are born without sight or hearing and utterly reliant on their mother for survival.

Puppies spend much of this period sleeping, nursing, and learning fundamental motor abilities like crawling.

2. Phase of Change (Lasts 2–4 Weeks):

• Puppies become more alert and aware when they open their eyes and ears.

• They begin to take an interest in their surroundings and engage with their littermates, laying the groundwork for future social and language development.

3. Beginning at the Third to Twelfth Week:

• This is a pivotal time for developing interpersonal skills. Puppies can benefit socially and emotionally from early socialization with a wide range of people, animals, and settings.

• The first steps of training can be taken, including as housebreaking and learning basic instructions like "sit."

4. Early Adolescence (Months 3-6):

• Teething begins around this time for puppies. For their comfort and the safety of your stuff, stock up on suitable chew toys.

• Their growth is quick, so consult your vet about making dietary adjustments.

• You should keep up with basic training and give your puppy lots of new experiences so that he or she grows up to be a well-rounded dog.

5. Late Childhood (age 6-18 months):

• At this age, Irish Terriers are considered to be teenagers. They may try to disobey you or push against your limits. Training should be consistent.

• They may become more physically active as they continue to develop physically.

• Maintain a steady and patient training regimen to help them through this difficult time.

6. By roughly 1-2 years of age, Irish Terriers often reach their full adult size and mature both physically and cognitively.

• Maintain routine veterinary checkups and reinforce training to keep them healthy.

7. Adulthood (Age 7+):

• Slowing down and dietary changes may be necessary as your Irish Terrier reaches old age.

The importance of routine veterinary examinations increases as pets age so that their health may be monitored and any age-related problems can be treated.

It's crucial to your Irish Terrier's development to give it the best care in terms of diet, exercise, and socializing. Consult with your veterinarian to develop a treatment strategy that takes into account your pet's age and unique traits. To guarantee a well-mannered and content adult dog, it's important to be patient and persistent with training.

Outside the Pale

Assuming you already know the fundamentals of training dogs and your Irish Terrier is well-behaved, you can move on to more sophisticated methods of development and enrichment. Some options for more advanced study and practice are listed below.

1. Advanced Instructions for Obedience:

• Improve your dog's self-control and attentiveness with advanced obedience training by teaching it more complex instructions like "stay," "leave it," "quiet," and "heel."

2. Training for Agility:

• Take your dog to an agility class or build a course at home. This might be a fun way to get some exercise and get to know one another at the same time.

3. Flyball, canine freestyle, dock diving, and obedience competitions are all great options. These activities put your dog to the test while providing you with hours of entertainment.

4. Training for a Trick:

• Rolling over, acting dead, and dancing are just a few of the fun and interesting things you may teach your Irish Terrier. Learning new tricks is a fun way to challenge your brain and may be a great conversation starter at parties.

5. The Nose Job:

• Involve your dog in scent exercises, such as tracking or finding concealed objects. Dogs have a highly developed sense of smell, and these games make use of that.

6. Dogs that can freestyle:

• Canine freestyle dancing is a fun activity in which you and your dog learn and perform dance routines to music. It's a fun and novel approach to connecting with your canine companion.

7. Instruction for Working or Therapy Dogs:

• If your dog has the correct temperament and skills, consider training them to become a service or therapy dog. These jobs typically need much education and training but pay very well.

8. Behavior Modification

• If your Irish Terrier has problems with anxiety, fear, or aggression, it's best to consult with a dog trainer or behaviorist. In order to deal with and control these problems, further education is essential.

9. Training without a Leash:

• In fenced dog parks and other safe settings, train your dog to walk without a leash. There must be complete faith and submission for this to work.

10. Day Hikes or Overnighters:

• Take your Irish Terrier camping, trekking, or backpacking if you're an outdoor enthusiast. These pursuits are great for your health and brain.

11. Complex Social Interactions:

• Keep exposing your dog to new experiences, including new people, animals, and places. This keeps their self-assurance and flexibility high.

12. Dogs competing in events:

• Participate in canine sports or competitions like obedience trials, agility trials, or conformation shows if your dog is of the suitable breed and temperament.

13. Tracking:

• Follow a scent trail with your Irish Terrier and other tracking activities. It's a mentally tough workout that activates their innate inclinations.

14. If you love dogs and want to meet other people who share your passion, you should join a canine sports or obedience club in your area.

Keep your dog's well-being and security as a top priority at all times. Dogs vary greatly in their interests and talents, therefore it's important to pick the activities carefully. You and your Irish Terrier should look forward to advanced training and activities since doing so will enhance your relationship.

Conclusion

Irish Terrier care entails familiarity with the breed's peculiarities, medical attention, obedience instruction, and mental enrichment. These dogs are great companions because of their high intelligence and lively personalities, but they only flourish when their individual needs are addressed.

The main points are summed up here.

- **Understanding the Breed**: Irish Terriers are noted for their energetic, confident, and friendly disposition. Responsible ownership requires familiarity with their background, appearance, and personality.

- Maintaining your Irish Terrier's health requires your attention to a number of factors, including regular veterinary treatment, correct nutrition, activity, grooming, and attention to unique breed-related health concerns.

• Obedience Training The cornerstone of having a well-mannered and secure Irish Terrier is teaching it basic obedience commands like sit, stay, and come. Training techniques based on positive reinforcement are advocated for.

• Engaging in cerebral exercises, puzzles, socialization, and interactive play with your Irish Terrier is essential for preventing boredom and ensuring a happy, well-rounded dog.

• Growth and Development Knowing how Irish Terriers develop from puppies to adults allows you to give your dog the best care possible.

• Further expand your Irish Terrier's life and strengthen your bond by engaging in more advanced training, activities, and even contests once they've mastered the basics.

By adhering to these rules, you can ensure that your Irish Terrier has a happy and healthy home life, where it can flourish and become a treasured family member. Always remember that each dog is unique, and it's crucial to personalize your care and training to your specific pet's needs and personality.

THE END